Natural High Blood Pressure Solutions

Lower Your Blood Pressure Naturally Using Diet And Natural Remedies Without Medication

MELODY AMBERS

Copyright © 2015 by Melody Ambers

All rights reserved. No part of this publication may be reproduced, distributed, or transmitted in any form or by any means, including photocopying, recording, or other electronic or mechanical methods, without the prior written permission of the publisher, except in the case of brief quotations embodied in critical reviews and certain other noncommercial uses permitted by copyright law

ISBN-13:978-1519757968

ISBN-10:1519757964

TABLE OF CONTENTS

Other Books By Melody Ambers 3
INTRODUCTION 1
PART 1: UNDERSTANDING BLOOD PRESSURE 3
    What Really Is Blood Pressure & High Blood Pressure? 3
    Who Develops High Blood Pressure 5
    Symptoms Of High Blood Pressure 6
    Causes Of High Blood Pressure 7
    The Damages Of High Blood Pressure 9
Part II: NATURAL WAYS TO LOWER BLOOD PRESSURE 13
    Diet And Nutrition 13
    The Salt Problem 17
    The Sugar Problem 22
    Fasting 23
Lifestyle Changes 25
    Hypertension and Obesity 25
    The Need For Exercise 25
    Reduce Your Alcohol Consumption 26
    Quit smoking 26
Mind-Body Approaches To Lower Blood Pressure 29

Meditation	29
Breathing Exercises	29
Relax With Music	30
Herbs& Supplements For High Blood Pressure	31
Herbal Homemade Recipes	36
Essential Oils For Blood Pressure	44
Conclusion	45

Other Books By Melody Ambers

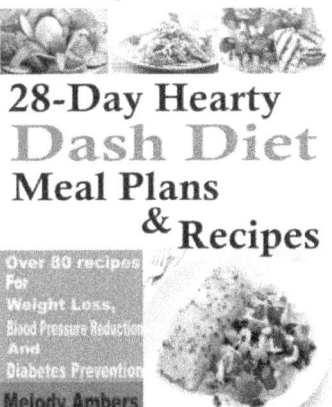

28-Day Hearty Dash Diet Meal Plans & Recipes: Over 80 recipes For Weight Loss, Blood Pressure Reduction And Diabetes Prevention

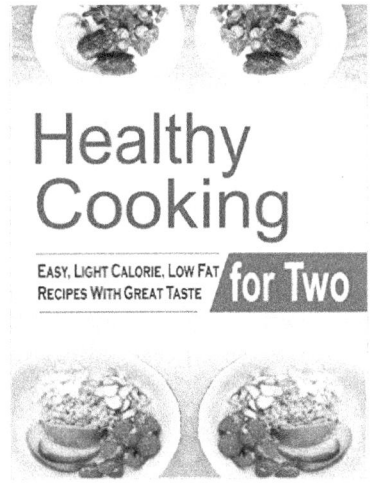

Healthy Cooking For Two: Easy, Light Calorie, Low Fat Recipes With Great Taste

Disclaimer

The information in this book is solely for informational purposes, not as a medical instruction to replace the advice of your physician or as a replacement for any treatment prescribed by your physician. The author and publisher do not take responsibility for any possible consequences from any treatment, procedure, exercise, dietary modification, action or application of medication which results from reading or following the information contained in this book.

If you are ill or suspect that you have a medical problem, we strongly encourage you to consult your medical, health, or other competent professional before adopting any of the suggestions in this book or drawing inferences from it.

This book and the author's opinions are solely for informational and educational purposes. The author specifically disclaims all responsibility for any liability, loss, or risk, personal or otherwise which is incurred as a consequence, directly or indirectly, of the use and application of any of the contents of this book.

INTRODUCTION

High blood pressure is the most prevalent medical condition on earth. The average American seems to be caught in the trendy lifestyle of fast food, soda and stress. The American heart Association estimates that 1 out of 3 Adult Americans has high blood pressure. This is about 67 million people, nearly 31% of the total population of the nation! This is alarming enough and even more alarming is the fact that most people who have high blood pressure are unaware of the situation and even when they do, they manage it poorly.

It is no longer advisable to put too much faith in the medical establishment to find a cure for this prevailing problem. Prescription drugs aren't reliable. A search in the drug store will bring out a plethora of prescription drugs and sadly, a dependable cure for blood pressure is not among them. Toxic, expensive drugs with their serious side effects cannot effectively lower blood pressure. A large number of patients are still being treated through this manner and their conditions have in no way improved. Rather, they also have to deal with side effects and the high cost of maintaining these expensive drugs. These drugs simply cover up the symptoms and ultimately truncate the quality of your life.

Despite all its associated consequences of strokes, kidney problems and heart diseases; to name just a few, high blood pressure is a preventable epidemic. The safest way to cure it is to remove the actual cause. The natural way to address it is to totally remove the poisons from the system which cause it. Diet, natural hormones, proven supplements, exercise, ending all bad habits and weekly fasting are the path to wellness. With natural medicines, diet and lifestyle, you will be able to address the core of your problems.

You can take proactive steps to manage your blood pressure. By enjoying an active, healthy lifestyle and observing a healthy balanced diet and of course, regular checks by the doctor, you can lower your elevated blood pressure and even avoid the risk altogether.

High blood pressure isn't a disease, but, if it is left unattended to, will worsen into one. This book highlights various ways to normalize your blood pressure naturally and enjoy the best of health!

Congratulations on your purchase!

PART 1: UNDERSTANDING BLOOD PRESSURE

What Really Is Blood Pressure & High Blood Pressure?
Blood Pressure

Blood and its circulation are crucial to sustain life. They provide the cells and organs of the body with vital nutrients and oxygen. They also eliminate waste and carbon dioxide. When blood is pumped, it exerts a measure of force on the walls of the arteries (these are the blood vessels that carry blood from the heart to the rest of the body). The measurement of this force is the blood pressure. Blood pressure is simply the force with which blood is circulated around the body.

Two forces, the systolic and the diastolic pressure, pump blood through our bodies. They are measured by reference to two different numbers. The systolic pressure represents the highest point of pressure that is measured while the heart beats or contracts. It is the higher of the two numbers. The diastolic pressure, the lower figure, is measured when the heart is resting between beats. It represents the low point of your blood pressure. Blood pressure is usually measured in millimeters of mercury and recorded as mmHg. The normal blood pressure reading of a non-stressed adult is 120/80 mmHg.

High Blood Pressure

High blood pressure occurs when too much pressure is exerted on the walls of your arteries, distorting it and causing extra stress on the heart. High blood pressure is medically known as hypertension. Blood pressure readings of 140/90 mm-Hg and higher on repeated measurements is considered hypertension.

Long-term hypertension will increase your risk of heart disease and stroke. If you have high blood pressure, your heart will work extra hard to pump blood through your body. The muscles of all healthy arteries are somewhat flexible. High blood pressure creates a force that will cause their walls to overstretch. This overstretching could lead to vascular scarring, tiny tears in the blood vessels. Plaque/ cholesterol and other cells will build up and this can cause blood clots. Additionally, the walls will gradually become weakened and since parts of the arteries have been deprived of fresh oxygenated blood due to blockage or plaque build up, heart attacks and strokes will occur if the blood pressure rises.

The main pressure point is from the heart; but, it is the arterioles, the smallest arteries that determine the amount of blood pressure in the blood vessels. To raise blood pressure, these arterioles constrict or narrow while they dilate or open up to lower it.

The body's activities determine the amount of blood pressure that is needed. Blood pressure is low when a person is at rest or asleep and higher when he is active or under stress. When at rest, the heart does not beat so fast to circulate blood but when you are exercising, you need more blood to carry oxygen to the muscles. As a result, blood pressure increases to meet this demand. Your heart then pumps faster to release more blood with each beat. When you are angry or frightened, for example, the adrenal glands pump out stress hormones known as adrenaline. These hormones makes the heart beat faster and harder, causing an increase in blood pressure and blood flow to the muscles.

Pre-hypertension is when the blood pressure is borderline high. It has a systolic reading of 120-139 and diastolic of 80-89.

The Blood Pressure Ranges are:

- Normal range: 120/80
- Pre-hypertension: 120-139/80-89
- High blood pressure (Stage 1): 140-159/90-99
- High blood pressure(Stage 2): 160 and above/100 and above

An elevated diastolic pressure is often more serious than an elevated systolic pressure because its effect are long-term and more severe as well. A higher blood pressure will cause more damages to the wall of the arteries.

Who Develops High Blood Pressure

High blood pressure affects both men and women of all social and economic groups. Nevertheless, age is a predominant factor. The older you get, the higher your pressures. Consequently, hypertension generally develops in adults between the ages of 35 and 50. These days, however, it is occurring more among children and youth. Rare cases have even been found in preadolescent children of between 3 and 13.

Some people are more prone to hypertension than others. These include:

- African-Americans: Studies have shown that blacks are twice as likely as whites to develop high blood pressure. Their cases have also been recorded to be more severe.

- People who have a family history of hypertension: there is a genetic basis for some hypertensive cases. Babies born to hypertensive parents are likely to have higher blood pressures or more variable blood pressures throughout childhood. They are also more likely to develop hypertension at an early age. But this is not always the case.

- People with diabetes:

- People who are overweight

Symptoms Of High Blood Pressure

High blood pressure in its mild or moderate form may not produce any symptoms for years. This is the reason it is aptly referred to as the silent killer. The majority of those who are affected do not know it until it is almost too late. This is due to its lack of symptoms or its remarked closeness to symptoms that might be considered normal or mild enough to conclude that nothing seriously could be wrong.

Then again, some 'lucky' people do suffer symptoms that show them all is not well with their body. For instance, a persistent unexplained nosebleed could suggest a high blood pressure problem. This is because the high blood pressure pumped around the body may rupture the weaker blood vessels in the nose. Similarly, dizziness, unexplained headaches, blurred vision, nausea are pointers to a high blood pressure problem. But, most of us are likely to pop an aspirin to alleviate a headache or pain than to see the doctor for a blood pressure check.

There are other more serious symptoms such as frequent fatigue, irregular heartbeats, breathing difficulties, ear buzzing, dyspepsia, confusion and inability to engage in serious work. High blood pressure that remains unchecked for years may lead to heart attacks, strokes or some serious organ damage or other disability conditions. In fact, high blood pressure is a problem with age so you will need frequent checks by your doctor as you grow older.

Causes Of High Blood Pressure

The causes of high blood pressure are in two categories: essential or primary hypertension and secondary hypertension. Primary hypertension has no single identifiable cause; it is associated with diet, environment, genetics, an irregular lifestyle including smoking, excessive intake of intoxicants and lifestyle factors, including a high salt intake, stress, inactivity and obesity. Primary hypertension affects a higher percentage of people; about 90% of people with high blood pressure. This is more dangerous because of its unidentifiable and silent nature: most people who have high blood pressure are not even aware of it.

Secondary hypertension is generally a result of other underlying and often serious medical conditions such as renal stenosis, tumors or liver disorders. It could also be a consequence of certain medications such as birth control pills. However, most people who are affected by the secondary level of hypertension are likely to be undergoing treatment for their medical conditions. Treatment for their elevated high blood pressure will likely be a part of their general treatment. Since this is identifiable, the high blood problem is more likely to be effectively controlled.

Primary Causes

Obesity Or Being Overweight

The heart of an overweight person works harder to pump blood around it, causing an increase in the pressure on the arterial walls. The bigger your body mass, the more blood is generated to supply the needed oxygen and nutrients.

Overweight people also face the risk of Sleep apnea, a condition where someone stops breathing for brief periods whilst asleep. This causes high blood pressure as well.

Genetics Or Family History

High blood pressure could be passed down from generation to generation. Therefore, if you have a family history of hypertension, chances are that you may have it.

Inactivity/ lack of exercise

Being inactive and ignoring exercises causes the heart to work harder in pumping blood around the body. Then again, an inactive person with a totally sedentary lifestyle is bound to be overweight.

Tobacco Use

Cigarettes and tobacco contain certain chemicals that can damage the blood vessel walls, consequently increasing the work of the heart in pumping blood around your body.

Excessive Alcohol Consumption

Excessive consumption of alcohol over a period of time can increase the risk of heart problems.

Stress

People who lead stressful life suffer from high blood pressure. Prolong stress causes the blood pressure to become permanently elevated and may not go away even after the stress is removed.

Sodium intake

Excessive sodium intake from salt could lead to fluid retention and ultimately an elevated blood pressure.

The Damages Of High Blood Pressure

High blood pressure puts every single blood vessel in the body, under increased pressure every minute of the day. Every vein, capillary and artery is overwhelmed and on the verge of breaking apart; whether you are at rest or at work. Definitely, this is bound to cause some sort of damage to the body. The truth is; if you suffer persistent high blood pressure, nowhere in your body is safe. High blood pressure increases your risk for stroke, heart attack, heart failure, vision loss, kidney disease, and metabolic syndrome. The most important organs of your body could give up at any time. Therefore, the only way to be safe is to check your blood pressure regularly.

The following are some problems that high blood pressure could cause to your body:

Heart Attacks And Cardiovascular Disease

High blood pressure aggravates any heart or artery problem. The majority of people who suffer their first heart attacks are usually high blood pressure sufferers as well. At the moment, the leading cause of death in the United States is heart attack, claiming two and half thousand people every day. High blood pressure can lead to several different fatal heart problems. The heart, being overwhelmed with the pressure of pumping an increased amount of blood to the body could just give up at any time. In its less serious form, it leads to an increasing level of heart failure, which if left unchecked, could become fatal. A heart, made enlarged by constant high pressure, will be unable to work efficiently. There may be other associated medical problems as well.

Strokes And Other Brain Problems

Strokes are the next most common cause of death in America. High blood pressure, if uncontrolled, could narrow the blood vessels in the brain or even damage them. This action may obstruct or rupture the blood vessels, thereby restricting the flow of blood to certain areas of the brain. The brain cells of that particular area will then cease to function. The affected person may die.

This is the reason why you should consult your doctor if you suffer constant persistent and severe headaches, blurred visions, dizziness, inextricably weakness or numbness as these could mean an imminent blood vessel failure in your head and an impending stroke caused by high blood pressure.

Other brain problems that high blood pressure could cause is dementia, particularly, vascular dementia. Once a part of the brain becomes damage due to irregular or erratic blood flow, the result is disorientation, memory loss and loss of speech. Unfortunately, it is often irreversible and the sufferer will become worse over time. High blood pressure also contributes to Alzheimer's, mental decline, senility and poor cognition.

Kidney Problems

The kidneys are the waste-removing organ; charged with the function of filtering blood to eliminate waste products from the body as urine, as well as returning nutrients and other useful substances to the body.

Persistent high blood pressure forces the kidneys to work harder. Eventually, the increased blood pressure may damage the kidney's tiny blood vessels and reduce the amount of blood that is available to it. After a while, the kidneys will be unable to filter the blood well. Protein may be excreted in the urine instead of being returned to the bloodstream and the waste products that should have been eliminated from the body will build up in the blood. This causes kidney failure.

Additionally, repeated kidney infections and inflammation can also cause high blood pressure. Kidneys help in controlling blood pressure by secreting rennin, a natural chemical. If the kidneys secrete an increased amount of rennin, the body will retain more salts. This will lead to an increase in the flow of blood and invariably, an increase in blood pressure.

Limbs And Eyes

Besides causing damage to your heart, kidneys and brain, high blood pressure can damage other areas of your body where there are blood vessels. Your eyes and your limbs are at risk of being damaged. This is the reason doctors often check your eyes once your blood pressure is increased. The capillaries, the thin blood vessels, at the back of the eyes will be checked to ascertain whether they have become enlarged, ruptured or suffer any other damage. If some damage is established, your eyesight will eventually be adversely affected in some way.

High blood pressure makes the heart become thicker and less able to do its job of pushing blood around the body effectively. This results in swollen ankles and limbs; and, as more blood accumulates in your lower legs and ankles, more serious problems like varicose veins and cellulitis will surface.

Mobility is a problem for high blood sufferers. They suffer leg cramps and painful ankle joints when they walk. This could also be signs of peripheral arterial disease, brought about by consistent narrowing of the arteries which in turn prevents sufficient blood from getting to the limbs.

Other Problems And Considerations

High blood pressure comes with other problems and considerations for both sexes. One of which is erectile dysfunction for men. High blood damages the arteries that carry blood to the penis. Consequently, the affected male will be unable to sustain an erection.

Also, some women suffer hypertension in pregnancy, especially during the last three months. In pregnancy, blood pressure levels are generally on the low side of normal (90–110/70–75). Blood pressure readings above 135-140/85–90 should be regarded as elevated and dealt with. Nevertheless, the condition is usually temporal and vanishes after the birth of the baby. But if the elevated blood pressure persists several weeks after delivery, you should consult your doctor.

High blood pressure is a serious problem for diabetes sufferers. If you are one, you should begin treatment as soon as possible. Diabetes hardens the arteries, making it difficult for them to pump blood to other organs of the body. As a diabetic, you are at higher risk of suffering strokes, heart problems and kidney diseases.

Another thing to keep in mind in terms of high blood pressure is hormone replacement therapy (HRT). Estrogen, a hormone that can increase blood pressure, is generally included in HRT. Consequently, you should check your blood pressure often whilst on HRT. Also, some birth control bills contain estrogen that can elevate blood pressure.

Part II: NATURAL WAYS TO LOWER BLOOD PRESSURE

Natural ways to lower blood pressure include good nutrition, healthy lifestyle habits, botanicals, herbs and nutritional supplements as well as mind-body techniques.

Diet And Nutrition
THE DASH DIET

Dash is an acronym that stands for Dietary Approaches to Stop Hypertension. It is a product of scientific research from the National Institutes of Health. It also has the support of the Heart, Lung and Blood Institute. Dash recipes simply entail the consumption of lots of fruits, vegetables, low-fat dairy products, whole grains, poultry, fish and nuts. Sugary beverages, red meats and sweets are featured in limited quantities. With the dash eating plan, cholesterol and saturated fat is limited while the focus is on the increase of the consumption of nutrients such as fiber, protein and minerals like calcium, potassium and magnesium.

Dash emphasises whole grains as your main staple. Eat at least 50% of it every day. Vegetables are emphasized as your secondary food. DASH menus that contains 2,300 milligrams of sodium helps to lower blood pressure and 1,500 milligrams of sodium in dash menus lowers it even further. This means the lower your salt consumption, the lower your blood pressure.

Although initially designed for individuals with hypertension, the DASH diet is presently recommended for anyone who wants to stay healthy. It is an established method to gain sound health and lose weight. It is the one-stop diet plan to help in managing diabetes.

For a complete meal plan on dash diet, get my book *28-Day Hearty Dash Diet Meal Plans & Recipes: Over 80 recipes For Weight Loss, Blood Pressure Reduction And Diabetes Prevention*

Mineral-Rich Foods To Lower Blood Pressure

If you want to lower your blood pressure, you will need to follow the DASH diet. Besides limiting sodium, the DASH diet promotes foods that are rich in magnesium, calcium and potassium. Potassium has been confirmed to lower blood pressure. These minerals are found in a variety of food sources. Therefore, it is best to eat a varied diet that is healthy and nutrient-rich. This will go a long way to prevent blood pressure problems.

If you are low in these minerals, the DASH diet will be of tremendous benefit to you. It is advisable to use food sources as opposed to supplements, to get maximum nutritional benefit.

Potassium:

Potassium is considered an effective high blood pressure treatment. It works by flushing out and cleaning the arterial walls. It also helps to remove excess sodium from the body.

It is found in:

- Various fruits such as such as bananas, apricots, prunes, avocado, oranges, cantaloupe, and kiwi.
- Dairy foods such as milk and yogurt.
- Vegetables including green beans, spinach, pumpkin, stewed tomatoes, winter squash sweet potatoes and dry peas and beans.

- All meats, including poultry and fish.

Calcium are in abundance in dairy foods, especially skim or low-fat varieties. Lower-fat products save calories and contain more calcium. Swiss chard and spinach contain lots of calcium. Others include:

- Tofu (prepared with calcium sulfate)
- Mackerel and salmon
- Milk, cheese and yoghurt

Magnesium is found in:

- Dry peas and beans including Lima and pinto.
- Greens such as okra, spinach, broccoli and Swiss chard.
- Pumpkin, sunflower and sesame seeds.
- Whole grains such as brown rice, millet and quinoa.
- Almonds and cashews.
- Halibut, scallops and salmon.
- Whole-grain cooked cereals and breads.

Fruit And Vegetables

Fruit and vegetables are rich in vitamins, minerals and fibre. They contain potassium as well, and you know that this can help in balancing out the negative effects of salt. This enables you lower your blood pressure.

Eat five portions a day. The following amounts represent a portion.

- Three heaped tablespoons of vegetables
- A dessert bowl of salad
- One tablespoon of dried fruit

- Three heaped tablespoons of pulses (such as beans, chickpeas and lentils)
- Two smaller fruits (apricots, plums, satsumas)
- One medium-sized fruit (banana, apple, pear, orange)
- One slice of one large fruit (pineapple, melon, mango)
- Two to three tablespoons of grapes or berries
- A glass (150ml) of vegetable or fruit juice

Not all veggies count. Plantains, yams, potatoes, cassava and sweet potatoes are all vegetables but they should not be counted towards your 5 a day portion. Still, add them as part of a healthy diet.

Vegetable juice, pulses and fruit juice could be counted as part of your 5 day portion; but, include them as just one portion irrespective of the quantity you drink or eat.

Getting The Best From Fruit And Vegetables

- Do not add salt to vegetables or sugar to fruit when you cook or serve them.

- Do not buy fruit and vegetable dishes that are sold with sauces. They usually contain lots of fat, sugar and salt.

- Make fruit smoothies with plenty of fresh fruit and low-fat milk or yoghurt.

- Eat a variety of fruit and vegetables. Each has its own different health benefits and will keep your meals interesting as well.

- Lightly steam or bake your vegetables to retain its vitamins and minerals. Do not boil. If you do, use very little water.

- Roast or grill vegetables for new tastes and flavors.

- Vegetables like carrot, cucumber, tomatoes, spinach, radish, onion and cabbage are best taken in their raw form.

The Salt Problem

The main ingredient in table salt is sodium. Sodium raises our blood pressure and increases the risk of heart disease and stroke. Too much salt consumption disrupts the balance of fluid in your body. When there is too much salt in the body, the body draws water from the surrounding tissues in a bid to flush it out. There is then a higher volume of liquid and the heart must now work harder to pump blood and this raises your blood pressure.

Most Americans eat twice as much salt as they need, about 3,400 milligrams of sodium daily. Ideally, a healthy adult require just 1 teaspoon of salt per day which is less than 2,300 milligrams of sodium (according to a 2010 Dietary Guidelines for Americans). It is best to limit your salt consumption to 1500-2000 mg daily. Children as well as the elderly, African Americans and those with high blood pressure need only 1,500 mg of sodium a day.

Only 6% of our salt intake comes from the table shaker. Most of the salt we eat is found in prepared food such as biscuits, breakfast cereals, bread and ready meals. To avoid unnecessary salt consumption, we must shop wisely and be cautious of the sodium levels in our diets.

Read Labels

Get into the habit of reading labels to see how much salt is contained in the food that you are about to buy. Labels may indicate the quantity of salt in each portion, pack or in every 100 g.

Some labels tell you how much sodium is contained in the food. Sodium is the leading chemical in salt, and 1g sodium = 21/2 grams of salt.

The ingredient list can also be helpful. If you check the ingredient list and salt is close to the top of the list, chances are that the food is likely to contain more salt.

Amount of salt per 100g	
0.3g or less	Eat plenty of these
0.3g to 1.5g	Eat small amounts occasionally
1.5g or more	Avoid these completely

How To Eat Less Salt

- Eat plenty of naturally low sodium foods such as fruits, vegetables, beans and peas.

- Do not add salt when cooking food; especially when cooking rice or pasta. Use unsalted butter or margarine. Things like stock cubes, soy sauce and curry powders should also be avoided.

- Get more flavors from seasonings like ginger, chilli, lime juice or lemon. Use different herbs and spices to flavor your food.

- Shop for canned foods that are labelled "reduced sodium", "no salt added" or "low sodium," but if they are unavailable, wash your beans and vegetables with water before you eat them. This will wash some of the salt away.

- Choose low- salt table sauces like mustard, pickles and ketchup as they often contain plenty of salt. Check the labels before making your purchase.

- Breakfast cereals and bread usually contain lots of salt. Therefore, check the labels in order to compare brands. In addition, compare salad dressings, frozen meals and soups to know the levels of sodium and opt for the ones with less sodium.

- If you buy pasta or rice that has a seasoning packet included in the package, reduce the sodium content by using only part of the packet.

- Avoid smoked meats and fish as much as possible because they contain lots of salt. Limit your consumption of processed foods as well, e.g. deli meats, bacon and hot dogs.

- You could try requesting for your meals to be made with less salt, if you are eating out. It's worth a try, especially if it is your favourite restaurant.

- Use a small quantity of low-sodium salt substitute if you really want a salty flavor. But check with your doctor first if you have diabetes or kidney problems.

- Reduce your consumption of luncheon meats such as bologna, processed turkey, corned beef, ham, pastrami and salami

- Don't be overly concerned about the precise amount of salt you eat. The recommended daily maximum is six grams a day, and the less you eat, the better for you.

- Search for low-salt recipe cookbooks in bookstores and on the internet. There are a number of them available.

- At first, your less- salt intake journey may seem difficult because your food will taste bland but with time, your taste buds will adjust.

Food On The Run? Do A Quick Sodium Check

The following are sodium levels in some single menu items gotten from some popular fast-food chains. Courtesy United Healthcare newsletter

Food Item	Amount Of Sodium	Recommended Daily	Recommended Daily For Adults With High Blood Pressure, Kids
Bacon, egg, cheese biscuit	1,160 mg	2,300 mg	1,500 mg
Crispy chicken sandwich	1,560 mg	2,300 mg	1,500 mg

Chicken quesadilla	1,210 mg	2,300 mg	1,500 mg
Quarter-pound burger with cheese	1,190 mg	2,300 mg	1,500 mg
Six-inch Italian sub sandwich	1,520 mg	2,300 mg	1,500 mg

The Sugar Problem

We eat more sugar than we need. Every year, Americans consume over 160 pounds of various sugars. Whether it's raw sugar, brown sugar, white sugar, corn syrup, fruit juice, fructose, dried fruit, molasses, agave, maple syrup cane syrup, honey, or any other kind of sugar, their negative effects on our health are the same. Even sugar substitute like stevia cannot be trusted.

Recent research has shown that high intake of sugar, particularly fructose, raises systolic by 6.9mm and diastolic blood pressure by 5.6mmHg in 8 weeks or more trial in duration. The study by open heart also pointed out that participants who consume at least 25% calories from added sugar are thrice likely to die from cardiovascular disease.

There is an established connection between sugar and metabolic syndrome, which includes insulin resistance, high cholesterol, excess weight and high blood pressure. Sugar consumption increases insulin levels; this triggers the nervous system, causing an increase in heart rate and consequently, blood pressure

You do not need sugar in your diet. Instead go on a whole grain based diet devoid of sugars or added sweets as best as you can. Avoid sugar substitutes like sucralose or stevia because they are just the same as regular simple sugars.

Fasting

Fasting helps you to eat less. Short-term fasting is especially good; you will hardly feel it as opposed to longer-term fasting which is more arduous but far more rewarding as well. You could fast once a day in a week from dinner to dinner. You could even do a 2-day monthly fast. You will feel much lighter and better.

Tips On How Manage High Blood Pressure With Dieting

Maintain a healthy body weight:

- Choose low -fat foods and eat smaller portions.
- Increase dietary fiber. Get 25- 35 grams of fiber every day.

Eat more foods high in potassium, fiber and magnesium:

- Eat 4-5 servings a day of whole fresh fruit & 5 daily servings of vegetables. ½ cup cooked or one cup raw= 1 servings.
- Include peas, nuts, dried beans and seeds about four times in a week for magnesium, potassium and fiber.
- Choose citrus fruit 3ce in a week for fiber and potassium.

Eat more foods that contain lots of calcium:

- Choose fat-free or low-fat cheese and yogurts. Use Lactaid or lactose-reduced milk if you are lactose intolerant.

Reduce caffeine:

- Choose decaffeinated tea, coffee and diet sodas.
- Do not take more than two caffeinated beverages daily even if you do have one.

- Do not take medications that contains caffeine

Drink enough fluids

- Drink at least eight cups of water every day.

Avoid These Foods:

– Trans-fats and Omega-6 fats: These fats, often found in package foods and meat increase inflammation and blood pressure.

–Sugar: High sugar consumption will increase your blood pressure.

– Caffeine: Too much caffeine can elevate blood pressure.

Lifestyle Changes

Hypertension and Obesity

You must lose weight to lower your blood pressure, if overweight. Obesity is a major cause of blood pressure problems. To stay slim and fit without necessarily being hungry, you will have to make better food choices such as we have discussed before.

By following the DASH diet, you will be able to lose weight and lower your risk of hypertension.

The Following Tips Should Help You Maintain A Healthy Body Weight:

- Keep a food diary. Check what you eat, the amount and when. By doing this, you will be on the right track to making changes and monitoring your progress.

- Portion sizes are important. Be mindful of these. Use smaller bowls, glasses and plates to make it easier for you to control portion sizes.

- Fill half of your plate with veggies at lunch and dinner. For dessert, take fruits. Fruit and vegetables have low calorie content and are rich in vitamins and minerals. They will also help you to satisfy your hunger.

The Need For Exercise

Physical exercise is important for promoting blood flow and strengthening heart function. It helps to lower blood pressure and aid weight loss as well. If you have high blood pressure, exercise can help to lower it but it could take up to 3 months to see a change. You will have to keep on doing the activity to notice a difference.

Engage in daily moderate cardiovascular exercise for at least 30 minutes. These include:

- brisk walking for 3 to 4 miles per hour
- racket sports like table tennis
- rowing (at 2-4 miles per hour)
- cycling (7-10 miles per hour)
- swimming

Before you begin an exercise program however, ask your doctor what amount of exercise as well as the type that will be suitable for you.

Reduce Your Alcohol Consumption

Alcohol narrows arteries, thereby increasing blood pressure. Limit your alcohol consumption. Healthy males should only take 2 drinks per day and no more, while women are advised to take just one drink a day. Anyone over 65 years however, should take only one drink in a day.

Quit smoking

Tobacco hardens the arteries and damages the blood vessel walls. If you have high blood pressure and you smoke, you are doing more harm to yourself. You will have to give up smoking. Begin by reducing the number of cigarettes that you smoke. Talk to your doctor as well to see how you can be helped.

Overview

S/n	Lifestyle Changes To Make	Blood Pressure Reduction	Notes
1	If overweight, lose weight	5-20 mmHg/ 10 kg wt. loss	Even little as 10 lbs can have significant effects
2	Limit salt in your diet	2-8 mmHg	Limit to less than 2400 mg/day (1 teaspoon)
3	Limit your intake of alcohol	2-4 mmHg	Limit to 2 drinks per day for men and 1 drink per day for women.
4	Exercise	4-9 mmHg	Aim for 30 to 40 minutes of physical activity every day, most days of the week.
5	Follow the DASH Diet	8-14 mmHg	
6	Do not use tobacco		Steer clear of first

			and second hand smoke and all tobacco products.

Mind-Body Approaches To Lower Blood Pressure

Mind-body approaches work by connecting a person's mind and body in order to promote health. Emotions such as anger, hostility and anxiety held on for too long can elevate high blood pressure and increase the risk of a heart attack.

Meditation

Meditation is a relaxation practice to soothe the mind and body. It involves clearing the mind and concentrating it on one thought. Examples include, yoga, Tai Chi and Qigong. People with mild high blood pressure who practiced meditation daily for 2-3 months experienced significant reductions in their blood pressure, had lower stress hormones levels, and were less anxious. A very recent study showed that participants who focused on a mantra, a repeated word or phrase, for 20 minutes daily for 16 weeks had their blood pressure lowered or improved. Yoga is a popular form of meditation. There is plenty of information about it on the internet. You can practice it in your home or join a local group or class.

Breathing Exercises

Controlled deep breathing is beneficial to blood pressure reduction. Deep breathing from the abdomen impacts on the nervous system, enabling the body to relax. There are many ways to do this, but one of the most effective methods is the Pavlov method of deep breathing. Pavlov is known for his 'conditioned reflexes' training which he successfully conducted on dogs by training their reflexes. This method teaches you to breathe deeply as a reflex reaction each time you are faced with a stressful situation. In fact, 15 minutes of slow breathing every day for 8 weeks has shown to bring about a considerable reduction in blood pressure. Aim for 5-6 breaths per minute.

To help you learn how to use your breath to reduce blood pressure, buy a biofeedback device, a small machine that measures bodily processes like breathing rate, muscle tension and heart rate. The device has a constant feedback that makes it possible to gain control over these measurements. Studies have shown that using a bio-feedback device after 8 weeks of treatment will lower blood pressure by 14 mmHg systolic and 8 mmHg diastolic.

There are many different types available on the internet or over the counter. One of which is the Resperate, an FDA approved device that can help you learn how to breathe deeply. It uses sound and a worn monitor around the chest to slow down breathing to 5-6 breaths per minute. Other biofeedback devices are Stress Eraser, EmWave Products, Resp-e-rate and Wild Divine products.

Relax With Music

Music, along with other natural hypertension remedies can alleviate high blood pressure. At the University of Florence in Italy, researchers asked 28 adults who were already treating their elevated blood pressure to listen to any soothing music. They were to choose from Indian, Celtic or classical music and listen to it for 30 minutes each day while breathing slowly. After only a week, the participants had reduced their average systolic reading by 3.2 points. Just one month later, the average readings were lowered to 4.4 points. Utilize the power of soothing music to eliminate stress and blood pressure.

Herbs & Supplements For High Blood Pressure

Herbs and spices contain antioxidant and anti-inflammatory properties to boost your body's health. Besides allowing you to lowering blood pressure naturally, herbs are low in calories and increase your food's medicinal value. It's a healthier and inexpensive alternative to taking prescription drugs and synthetic supplements so improve your heart and general health with herbs.

Herbs can be used whole. You can mix them up with your salads, soups, meat, fish and vegetable dishes or as a supplement. Whichever way you decide to go, be sure to consult your doctor first. Used in large quantities, certain herbs may cause unpleasant side effects.

Cardamom

Cardamom is a popular South Asian seasoning. A study to investigate its health effects showed that participants who took powdered cinnamon everyday for many months saw considerable reductions in the readings of their blood pressure. For best results, use cardamom seeds or powder in stews, soups and pastries.

Basil

Basil is a tasty herb that is used to cook various dishes. It has been proven to lower blood pressure briefly. For this reason, add some fresh basil to your meals such as soups, salads, casseroles and pastas. You could grow your own fresh herbs by keeping a small pot in your kitchen garden.

Garlic

Ignore the effect it will have on your breath, garlic is a wonder when it comes to helping to lower blood pressure. Garlic contains allicin, a substance with antioxidant, antibacterial, lipid lowering and, wonderfully, anti-hypertension properties. This pungent seasoning will cause your blood vessels to relax and dilate, enabling blood to flow easily and ultimately reducing blood pressure.

To use, add it fresh to several recipes of choice. You could roast it first to reduce the strong flavor or purchase in supplement form. Use garlic powder instead of salts in your recipes.

It can be infused in oil, added to your diet or used as a tincture or capsule. Do not heat beyond 130 degrees if cooking because it will reduce its potency.

Cats-Claw

This is a traditional Chinese herbal medicine that has been used to treat hypertension for many years. Studies have shown that it can help to reduce blood pressure by working on your cells' calcium channels. Cat claws are available in several health food stores in supplement forms.

Cinnamon

Cinnamon is delicious seasoning so you can add it easily to your daily diet to reduce your blood pressure readings. Cinnamon prevents heart disease and it is also helpful for people with diabetes. Simply sprinkle on your oatmeal, breakfast cereal and coffee. For dinner, add to your stews, curries and stir-fries for optimum health and flavor.

Celery Seed

The herb, Celery seed is used to season stews, casseroles, soups, and other flavorful dishes. although Celery has been used to treat hypertension in China for a long time, studies also shown that it may be effective. You can use the seeds to lower blood pressure, but you can also juice the whole plant. Celery is a diuretic, which may help explain its effect on blood pressure

Cayenne Pepper

Cayenne pepper is a potent vasodilator, this means it expands and dilates the blood vessels, consequently improving blood flow. This relives pressure on the arterial walls. Take 1 teaspoon in a glass of warm water every day to lower your blood pressure. If too hot for you, take cayenne pepper capsules.

Hibiscus

Hibiscus acts as a diuretic. It draws sodium from the bloodstream, thereby reducing the pressure on the arterial walls. Interestingly, it can also act like Angiotensin-converting enzyme (ACE) inhibitors. ACE inhibitors are group of medicines that help to relax blood vessels, lower blood volume and decrease blood pressure. They work by inhibiting the growth of a natural chemical, the angiotensin-converting enzyme, which helps to regulate blood pressure and fluid balance. ACE inhibitors work best when used in combination with diuretics rather than on their own.

Watermelon

Watermelon contains L-citrulline, an amino acid, which has been confirmed to lower blood pressure. According to the American Journal of Hypertension, the Florida State University conducted a research on hypertensive participants and concluded that L-citrulline was responsible for reduction and normalization of the participants' elevated blood pressure. It is advisable to take1 to 2 cups of fresh watermelon in the morning.

Coconut Water

Coconut water contains potassium and magnesium. It is found inside the shell of coconuts. It has been reported to help lower blood pressure by a number of people. Studies have also shown that it affects systolic blood pressure.

Fish Oil

Fish oil (particularly essential oil omega-3) can help to reduce blood pressure for many hypertension sufferers. Heart transplant patients have been given fish oil, after a transplant, to lower the risk of hypertension. It is advisable to go for high quality liquid fish oil taken in orange juice to the pills.

Olives

Oil made from olives helps to reduce blood pressure. Studies have confirmed that daily use of the olive oil up to 40 grams helps to lower the blood pressure of hypertensive patients by 50 percent. A substance, polyphenols, contained in extra-virgin olive oil enabled the considerable reduction of blood pressure.

Dark Chocolate

Dark chocolate contain flavanols, which enhances the elasticity of blood vessels. In one study, 18% of participants who ate dark chocolate everyday had their elevated blood pressure lowered. Take ½ ounce of dark chocolate daily with at least 200 mg of cocoa phenols. This amount helps to reduce blood pressure.

Coenzyme Q10

Studies have showed that Coenzyme Q10 lowers blood pressure by about 17 mmhg over 10 mmhg. The antioxidant, required for energy production, dilates blood vessels. Take 60 to 100 mg supplement three times daily but check with your doctor first.

Hawthorn

Hawthorn is rich in flavonoids, which helps different types of heart diseases, including the risk of hypertension. Hawthorn has been confirmed to lower blood pressure modestly and to treat congestive heart failure with its active ingredient, proanthocyanidins. It herbs has been used by Traditional herbal practitioners for many years. flavonoids helps in widening of the blood vessels, which in turn helps to reduce blood pressure. Hawthorn can be enjoyed in the form of a tea or "balls". See recipe in the next chapter.

Herbal Homemade Recipes

Here are homemade recipes that have been tested by many people to lower blood pressure. There are quite a number of them. Pick a few and you just might be among the many that they have worked for.

Cayenne Pepper Mix

1 teaspoon of cayenne pepper

½ cup of warm water

Combine and drink immediately.

Lemon Juice Mix

Juice of ½ of 1 lemon

Warm water

Combine and take every 2 hours.

Fenugreek Seeds Mix

1 teaspoon of fenugreek seeds

 Combine with water and take every morning and evening for 10 to 15 days.

Honey/Onion Juice

Equal part pure honey

Equal part onion juice

Combine and take 2 tablespoons daily for 2-3 days.

Store in an airtight container and refrigerate.

Amla/Milk Mix

1 teaspoon of amla (Indian gooseberry extract) mixed with milk

Take mixture every morning and evening

Coconut Water

8 ounces fresh, organic coconut water

Directions

Drink 1 to 2 times daily, mornings alone or morning and evenings if you drink twice daily.

Mint Tea For High Blood Pressure

1/4 cup fresh mint leaves

1/4 cup dried chrysanthemum flowers

2 tablespoons cassia seeds

5 cups of water

Combine and boil for 20 minutes. Strain and drink 3 cups of tea per day.

Vinegar & Honey

Honey helps to lower blood pressure. Vinegar alkalizes the body.

Ingredients

8 ounces of warm water

1 teaspoon honey

1 tablespoon apple cider vinegar

Directions

Mix them all together and drink first thing in the morning. Drink regularly.

Ginger

Make ginger tea with 1/2 to 1 teaspoon of powdered ginger

Ginger-Cardamom Tea

What You Need

1 teaspoon of cardamom pods

1 teaspoon of cinnamon powder

2 to 3 teaspoons of honey

1/2 cup of milk

2 teaspoons minced fresh ginger or 1/2 teaspoon ginger powder

1 teabag or 1½ tablespoons black tea

1/2 cup of water

Mortar and pestle

Directions

1. Release the oil in the cardamom by crushing them. Combine all ingredients, except for the honey, in a saucepan and bring to a boil.

2. Simmer for 6 to 9 minutes until a rich caramel brown color is achieved. Add honey, stir and strain into a mug.

3. Drink 1-2 times daily.

Celery Juice

A very popular and effective Chinese folk remedy for lowering blood pressure

8-ounce glass of fresh celery juice

Drink every morning for 1 to 3months until blood pressure normalizes.

Blueberry Syrup

Blueberries are rich in the flavonoid quercetin. For an extra heart healthy kick, add in elderberries as well.

What You Need

4 tablespoons each of dried blueberries and elderberries or 8 tablespoons of dried blueberries

1 cup of honey

4 cups of water

A strainer

A pot

A glass jar with an airtight lid

Directions

1. Combine the berries and water and simmer over low heat. Keep simmering until the liquid lessens by half.

2. Strain and pour back the liquid into the pot. Add honey and stir to blend well.

3. Heat the berry juice and honey over medium-high heat for 20 minutes to achieve thicker syrup. Leave as it if you prefer it thin.

4. Pour into a bottle, label and refrigerate for 3 to 4 weeks. Take 1 teaspoon two times daily

Herb Pillow

Stuff pillow with split peas, lentils and mung beans and sleep on it.

They help to lower blood pressure.

Cucumbers

Cucumber is a natural diuretic; therefore, it will assist in hydrating your body and to lower blood pressure.

Eat 2 fresh cucumbers daily for 2 weeks, or until your blood pressure improves.

Relax Lower Limbs Swelling

To relax and reduce swelling in your lower limbs caused by high blood pressure, soak your lower legs and ankles in a bowl of warm water for 10-15 minutes several times a day.

Hibiscus Sip

<u>What You Need</u>

1 to 2 teaspoon of dried hibiscus

1 cup of fresh hot water

Lemon or honey

1 to 2 cinnamon sticks (optional)

<u>Directions</u>

1. add the hibiscus and cinnamon sticks (if using) to boiling water. Let it steep for 5 minutes.

2. Add lemon or honey to taste. Drink 2 to 3 times daily.

3. Make as iced tea during the hot summer days.

Hawthorn Recipe

<u>What You Need</u>

4 tablespoons of powdered hawthorn berry

½ to 1 tablespoons of cinnamon powder

Raw honey

Carob or cocoa powder

Water

<u>Directions</u>

1. Combine the hawthorn powder and cinnamon in a bowl, mixing well.

2. Add enough honey and water moderately to make a paste. Add carob powder or cocoa powder to thicken the mixture until it forms dough. Roll into tiny balls like the size of the index fingernail.

3. Place on a cookie sheet, set oven to about 150 degrees Fahrenheit and dry. Store in a glass jar and in a cool place.

Epsom Salt

The Epsom Salt High Blood Pressure Drench

The Epsom salt contains magnesium which helps to lower blood pressure. The Epsom salt drench is highly effective because of the concentrated solution that is left on the skin. Regular use of this treatment can lower high blood pressure. Desired results can become noticeable a week after continued treatments.

<u>What To Do</u>

1. Dissolve 2 oz. of Epsom salt in 1 a quart of warm water.

2. Take a hot bath or shower to help open pores. Do this every evening.

3. After the shower or bath, pour the solution slowly over your whole body and as far as you can, to cover each part.

4. Let it stay on your body for 1-2 minutes then pat dry body with a towel. Do not rinse it off. This remedy helps to lower blood pressure.

Baking Soda

Seems ridiculous? However, as cheap and simple as baking soda is, it is effective in the reduction of hypertension. Baking soda is a powerful pH booster, spiking your body's pH level

Ingredients & Directions

1/8th of 1 teaspoon of baking soda

2 tablespoons of apple cider vinegar

Combine ingredients in 1 glass of water.

Take two times daily.

Essential Oils For Blood Pressure

Lavender, clary sage, frankincense and ylang ylang are very effective essential oils that help to lower blood pressure. They dilate arteries, act as antioxidants to lower oxidative stress and also decrease emotional stress.

Lavender

One of the most versatile oils, lavender has antiviral and antibacterial properties. It is relaxing and uplifting, helping to balance hormones in women and generally reducing the stress hormones in the body.

Uses

- To relax the body and improve sleep, rub on neck in the evenings.
- To restore the body after a long day, add a few drops to your bath.
- Diffuse in the air to improve mood and relax.
- Use topically on neck to lower cholesterol& blood pressure or take as supplement.

Ylang-ylang & Clary-Sage

1 drop Ylang-ylang

2 drops of Clary-Sage

Place these 3 drops on a tissue and inhale.

Conclusion

Although hypertension is prevalent, it is preventable. The first step is to have your blood pressure checked. You could see your doctor for this, or you could invest in a home blood pressure monitoring device. This way, you get to check your blood pressure regularly.

If you find out that you do have hypertension, you now have the information with which to use to address it. If you are obese or overweight, you will have to do something about it while treating your hypertension. The most important thing is that you will have to do something about your high blood pressure because it will not just disappear on its own.

Begin by isolating the cause of your hypertension and taking quick and effective steps to address it. This should be done as naturally as possible, to avoid the harmful effects of chemical-based pharmaceutical drugs as pointed out in the introduction.

Hypertension is a silent killer, remember that. It is a totally unnecessary epidemic. So take the necessary action NOW!

CPSIA information can be obtained
at www.ICGtesting.com
Printed in the USA
LVHW092336190421
684976LV00005B/276